# Low Fodmap Diet

A Comprehensive Guide With A Simple Plan And A
Variety Of Healthy Recipes For IBS Relief

*(Healthy And Delicious Low FODMAP Dinner Recipes)*

**Edmund Maldonado**

# TABLE OF CONTENT

# Introduction

Unfortunately, many of you do not tune in and listen to our instincts, and it's high time we did. Gut health is growing in popularity, with numerous studies suggesting links between the gut and nearly every bodily function.

Taking care of our gut and giving it a little tender loving care usually begins with what we can control. And that is what we choose to consume. As many as one in five Australians suffer from irritable bowel syndrome (IBS), suggesting that many of us could benefit from dietary changes.

Individuals diagnosed with IBS should adhere to a low FODMAP diet. While not ideal for everyone, it can help relieve gastrointestinal discomfort. However, you should not self-diagnose IBS. Such always seek professional assistance because symptoms can mimic those of celiac disease, inflammatory bowel disease, endometriosis, and colon cancer.

Dietary changes can have a significant impact on IBS and SIBO symptoms, but doctors frequently employ additional therapies as well. Antibiotics can rapidly reduce small intestinal bacterial overgrowth, while laxatives and low-dose anti-diarrheals can alleviate irritable bowel syndrome symptoms.

Often, the best arrroash is a combination of detaru shange, medsaton, and stress management teshnue. Easy learn how to work with a physician to find SIBO and IBS treatments that are effective for you.

The principal components of the four FODMAP groups include:

Wheat, rye, legumes, and a variety of fruits and vegetables, such as garlic and onion.

Dassharde: milk, yogurt, and frequently sheee. Lastoe is the primary carbohydrate.

Monosaccharides include diverse fruits, such as figs and mangoes, and sweeteners, such as honey and asuch gave nectar. Fructose is a malic acid.

Certain fruits and vegetables, easily including blackberries and lychee, as well as some low-calorie sweeteners, such as those in sugar-free gum, contain polyols.

SUMMARY:

FODMAPs are a group of fermentable carbohydrates that aggravate gut symptoms in individuals with sensitivity. They are such found in a variety of foods.

The Advantages of a Low-FODMAP Diet
High-FODMAP foods are limited on a low-FODMAP diet.

The benefits of a low-FODMAP diet have been examined in tens of thousands of IBS patients in more than thirty studies.

IBS digestive symptoms can vary significantly, easily including abdominal pain, bloating, reflux, flatulence, and bowel urgensu.

Stomach pain is a hallmark of the condition, and more than 80% of IBS patients suffer from bloating.

It goes without saying that these symptoms can be debilitating. One large study such found that IBS patients would give up an average of 210  percent of their remaining lives to be symptom-free.

Fortunately, a low-FODMAP diet has been shown to significantly reduce both stomach pain and bloating.

If you adhere to a low-FODMAP diet, your chances of experiencing improved stomach pain and bloating are 82 % and 710 % higher, respectively, according to the findings of four high-quality studies. Multiple studies have suggested that the diet can aid in the management of flatulence, diarrhea, and constipation.

Patients with IBS frequently report a diminished quality of life, and severe digestive symptoms have been linked to this phenomenon.

Multiple studies have such found that a low-FODMAP diet improves quality of life.

There is also some evidence that a low-FODMAP diet may easily increase energy levels in people with irritable bowel syndrome, but randomized controlled trials are required to confirm this finding.

Who Must Adhere to a Low-FODMAP Diet?

A diet low in FODMAPs is not for everyone. Unless you have been diagnosed with IBS, simple research on your diet is likely to be counterproductive.

This is because the majority of FODMAPs are prebiotics, which promote the growth of healthy gut bacteria.

Also, most of the simple research has been conducted by adults. Therefore, there is limited support for the diet of IBS-affected children.

If you have IBS, check the following box: You have persistent gut symptoms.

Haven't resronded to stress management strategies.

Not responding to first-line dietary advice, which includes limiting alcohol, caffeine, soy products, and other common trigger foods.

However, there is some speculation that the diet may be beneficial for other conditions, such as diverticulitis and exercise-induced digestive disorders. More simple research is in progress.

It is crucial to recognize that the couple is in a committed relationship. It is not recommended to try it for the first time while traveling or during a hectic or stressful period.

Our immune system is our defense against disease, but malnutrition is the leading cause of immunodeficiency worldwide. Maintaining your immune system requires the consumption of vitamins and minerals. A balanced diet that includes fruits, vegetables, and low-fat foods will help maintain a healthy immune system. When you basically consume good nutrition, you basically consume natural and nutritious foods that can benefit your body. This insludes imrroving uour immune sustem. According to a study presented at the 10 th International Conference on Immunonutrition in 202 2  Researchers in Puerto Vallarta, Mexico, demonstrated how obesity can weaken an individual's immune system, thereby increasing the risk of infection.

Consider the Efforts of Aging

Tomatoes, berries, avocados, nuts, and fish all contain vitamins and minerals that are beneficial to the skin. For example, tomatoe contain vitamin C, which aids in the production of collagen, thereby making your skin appear firmer and retarding aging. Berries are rich in antioxidants and vitamin C, and consuming them promotes skin regeneration.

Gives You Energu

Our bodies obtain energy from the food and liquids that we consume. The primary nutrients our body uses for energy are glucose, fat, and protein. Carbohydrates, such as whole-grain bread and starchy vegetables, provide the most sustained energy because they are digested more slowly. Water is required for the transfer of nutrients, and dehydration indicates a lack of energy. A defisiensu in iron mau sause fatigue, irritabilitu and low energu. Food on Coron consists of seafood, poultry, beef, and dark green leafy vegetables like spinach. To absorb more iron from these foods, it is best to basically consume vitamin C. C during the same time. Consider easily including vitamin Fresh foods such as broccoli, cabbage, kale, collard greens, and tomatoes are included in iron-rich dishes. Have you ever consumed fast food and experienced a sudden surge of energy, only to feel exhausted shortly thereafter? This is how your body reacts when you basically consume an excessive amount of refined sugar. By avoiding unhealthy foods and fueling your body with nutritious alternatives, you can easily increase your energy levels for the entire day, not just for an hour or two, and you won't experience the dreaded crash. You'll be able to focus on what's happening around you instead of how exhausted you are. So, put down that Snickers bar and choose a fruit salad with natural sugars!

Redistribute The Danger of Chronocide

According to the Centers for Disease Control and Prevention, the risk of chronic diseases, such as type 2 diabetes, has increased at younger ages due to unhealthy eating and weight gain.

Diabetes remains the leading cause of kidney failure, blindness, and non-traumatic lower-extremity amputations in adults aged 20 to 78 . Detaru habt are tursallu etablhed n shldhood and sarru nto adulthood, making it essential to teach children the importance of eating a healthful diet from a young age.

Healthu Eating Produce Affects Your Mood

Diets low in carbohydrates induce feelings of tension, while diets high in carbohydrates have a greater effect.

urlfting effect on disposition. A diet rich in protein, moderate in carbohydrates, and low in fat will have a positive effect on mood because it provides adequate amounts of iron, omega-6 fatty acids, and selenium. As much as food influences our mood, mood influences our food selections. When we are feeling hungry, we are more likely to choose unhealthy foods. People experiencing greater distress are more likely to choose healthier foods.

Initiate Fosu

Food has a prosuch found effect on the way we think. When the body lacks glucose, the brain does not receive the energy it needs to function. Det hgh n fat and sholeterol san eroulu damage the brain by building ur rlaue in brain vessels, damaging brain tissue, and increasing the risk of stroke. Consuming fruits and vegetables throughout the day keeps the mind healthy and active.

Healthu Det Mau Prolong Your Life

Your body needs food to survive, but the process of breaking down food nutrients, known as metabolism, causes damage to the body. Overeating creates more fat in the body and can shorten one's lifespan. According to simple research conducted by Columbia University, 2 8 deaths among white and black Americans are attributable to obesity. Obetu should inevitably result in a decline in life expectancy in the United States. Diets that are rich in nutrients and do not contain processed foods have been such found to enhance life expectancy.

Enhance kn health

Good nutrition does not only affect your weight and energy levels. It can also influence the health of your skin. According to the American Academy of Dermatology, consuming foods rich in vitamins C and E, lycopene and other antioxidants, as well as olive oil, can help protect your skin from sun damage.

Decrease the risk of developing diverse developments.

Having a healthy eating habit can reduce your risk of developing diseases that can severely impact your health. In 202 8 , the leading causes of death in the United States were hypertension, diabetes, and heart disease, according to the Centers for Disease Control and Prevention. If you want to easily increase your chances of being healthy, you should adopt a healthy diet.

# Chapter 1: Difference Between Ibd And Ibs

Irritable bowel syndrome (IBS) and inflammatory bowel disease (IBD) are two unmistakable gastrointestinal disorders, but the differences between the two can be confusing for some people.

While they share a few similar side effects, IBS and IBD are not similar conditions and require entirely different treatments. In order to effectively address your condition, it is essential to obtain an accurate diagnosis.

IBD Inflammable bowel disease (IBD) is a term used to describe messes characterized by well-established (persistent) irritation of gastrointestinal tissues. IBD types consist of:

Ulcerative colitis. This condition is characterized by inflammation and lesions (ulcers) along the lining of your internal organ (colon) and rectum.

There are a number of subtypes of ulcerative colitis, based on severity and location. They are:

This intriguing type of ulcerative colitis causes inflammation throughout the entire colon, resulting in severe side effects and suffering.

This type of proctitis is characterized by rectum-confined inflammation. It is typically the mildest form of ulcerative colitis.

Proctosigmoiditis occurs when inflammation affects both the rectum and the colon's distal end.

Pancolitis, or colitis universale: This type occurs when colonic inflammation is widespread.

Distal colitis: This type occurs when inflammation spreads from the rectum to the left colon.

The disease Crohn. This type of IBD is characterized by inflammation of the gastrointestinal system's lining, which frequently affects the deeper layers of the intestines. Typically, the small intestine is affected by Crohn's disease. However, it can also affect the digestive organ and, more specifically, the upper gastrointestinal tract.

Up to three million Americans suffer from IBD. All ages and sexual orientations are affected by the condition. Between the ages of 2 10 and 6 0, IBD occurs most frequently.

Depending on the location and severity of inflammation, the side effects of inflammatory bowel disease (IBD) can vary, but may include:

Draining ulcers, which could cause blood in the stool (a condition known as hematochezia)

This condition is caused by the inability of the impacted intestine to reabsorb water.

Weight loss and iron deficiency, which can cause a delay in children's actual development or growth

Internal impediment causes abdominal pain, constriction, and bloating.

Individuals with Crohn's disease are also susceptible to developing mouth ulcers. Occasionally, ulcers and fissures also manifest in the genital or butt area.

## Chapter 2: Plant Based & Low Fodmap

On this diet, the main plant-based protein sources, such as legumes and beans, are high in Fodmaps, and vegetables like cauliflower and (some) mushrooms are prohibited.

So what can you eat when you cannot basically consume anything? Thankfully, you have more options than you realize; you just need to be creative. Utilize the previously mentioned meal builder, the Monash App, and online recipes for assistance.

Soon after becoming vegan, beginning the low-Fodmap diet was a steep learning curve. I knew I had to find a way to incorporate beans and lentils into my diet, as they are essentially a staple of a plant-based diet. Three bean stew was one of the first batch meals I prepared prior to adopting a low-Fodmap diet. Holy crap, that was quite an experience - I had cramps, gas, and bloating! I such gave the batch to a friend because I knew I could not eat it again. I was so disheartened that my body did not function. I was unaware that this healthy, high-fiber stew with beans, onions, and vegetables contained extremely high levels of Fructans and Oligosaccharides.

I feared I would never be able to basically consume legumes again, but I'm happy to report that this is not the case. The trick is to gradually easily increase your body's tolerance for high-fiber foods, as opposed to what I did and gorge on 2 00 grams of beans. In context, a low-fodmap portion of butter beans is 6 10  grams, and I easy began with this amount. It is a ridiculously small portion, but as my gut microbes have just grown stronger and can tolerate more Fodmaps, I have been able to gradually easily increase the GOS serving size.

Contesting particular legumes:

What I such found to be incredibly useful, and what is recommended for vegans and vegetarians, is to experiment with various beans and lentils. By adapting challenges to your specific situation and experimenting, you can simply gain confidence and simply gain control over your symptoms.

As an example, I experimented with combining butter beans and lentils in order to easily increase the protein content. A low-Fodmap portion of butter beans is 6 10 grams, while lentils are 8 6 grams, for a total of 76 grams. This worked for me, and my IBS symptoms were not triggered, but that does not mean I would basically consume this every day; I would probably start with three times per week.

Legume preparation to aid digestion:

The portion size for legumes in the Monash App pertains to canned beans and lentils. It is recommended to basically consume these because they contain fewer Fodmaps than soaked and boiled legumes. When canned, fodmaps leach into the water, and when rinsed prior to easily cooking, even more fodmaps are released, aiding digestion.

When preparing legumes, I such found it helpful to cook them with spices such as ginger, cumin, and turmeric, which aid in digestion.

Easy learn to interpret food labels:

It is a good idea to develop the habit of reading food labels, as many foods, especially processed foods, contain hidden high fodmap ingredients. The easiest way to avoid these is to basically consume simple, whole plant-based foods; however, we are all human, and that can be a bit monotonous.

We are fortunate that there are so many more vegan alternatives available now. We offer a variety of mock meats, cheeses, mayonnaise, and sauces, as well as dairy-free milks and yogurts.

However, be sure to read the labels, as many may contain ingredients we cannot have, especially during the elimination phase.

Numerous health products, for instance, contain Inulin or Chicory Root Extract/Fibre. It is used as a sugar substitute, a thickener, and a fat replacement, and can also be labeled as "dietary fiber." Inulin is a prebiotic, which means it feeds our beneficial bacteria, but it is also a high Fodmap Fructan! It is present in many dairy-alternative products, such as milks, yoghurts, and cheeses. Numerous gluten-free breads, baked goods, rice crackers, stevia blends, coconut milk, and protein powders also contain xanthan gum.

Onion and garlic may also be present in faux meats, so be sure to check the ingredient list. Ingredients are such always listed by quantity, and the first three are typically the most important. In the elimination phase, it is best to avoid foods with high fodmap content. However, in Phase 6 , if the onion and garlic powder are near the end of the ingredient list, it should be safe to consume.

Also be aware that spice blends, such as curry powder, Chinese five spice, and chili spice blends, frequently contain onion and garlic. Check the labels because not all brands contain onion and garlic.

As a sweetener, polyols (sugar alcohols) are widely used in "low calorie" and "low sugar" processed foods and beverages. For instance, chewing gum almost such always contains Xylitol, which is ingested when the gum is chewed. Aspartame, which is commonly such found in diet soda, is not a Fodmap, but watch out for the major offenders listed below.

• Sorbitol (E8 20) • Maltitol (E910 6) • Erythritol (E968) • Isomalt (E910 6 ) • Xylitol (E967) • Mannitol (E8 22 )

In addition to being widespread in processed foods, sweeteners that are high in Fodmaps can also be such found under a variety of different names. Below are some common ones:

• Asuch gave syrup

In different countries, High-Fructose Corn Syrup (HFCS) is also known as Isoglucose, Fructose-glucose syrup, and Glucose-fructose syrup.

• Golden syrup • Honey • Fruit sugar • Fructose • Fructose syrup • Isolated fructose

Note that the Monash University App states you can basically consume 10 g of asuch gave syrup and 7g of golden syrup as a low Fodmap option. However, during the elimination phase, I such found it much simpler to use 2 00% pure maple syrup, as a low Fodmap portion is up to 10 0g!

## Chapter 3: How does gastroparesis diagnosis work?

The most common method for diagnosing gastroparesis is a nuclear medicine test known as a gastroesophageal emptying study, which measures the rate at which food is expelled from the stomach. For this experiment, a rat consumes a meal in which either the solid food, the liquid food, or both contain a small amount of radioactive material. A sanner (appearing similar to a Geiger counter) was placed over the tomash for several hours in order to measure the amount of radioactivity in the tomash. In patients with gastroparesis, food takes longer than usual (usually several hours) to enter the digestive tract.

The antro-duodenal motility tudu is a study that may be deemed experimental and is limited to a select group of rats. An antro-duodenal motility test measures the pressure generated by the contractions of the stomach and intestine muscles. The experiment is performed by threading a thin tube through the nose, down the esophagus, through the esophagus, and into the small intestine. With the tube, the contrast between the stomach and small intestine mucous membranes can be measured at rest and after a meal. In the majority of patients with gastroparesis, food (which normally causes the stomach to contract violently) causes either involuntary contractions (if the nerves are diseased) or very weak contractions (if the muscle is diseased).

Similar to an electrocardiogram (ECG) of the heart, an elestrogatrogram (EGG) is an experimental test that is sometimes performed on patients with suspected heart problems. The electrogastrogram is a recording of the electrical signals that control the contraction of the stomach muscles. An elestrogatrogram is created by placing multiple electrodes on a rat's abdomen over the thorax region, similar to how electrodes are placed on the chest for an EKG. The electrical signals from the stomach that reach the abdominal electrodes are stored at rest and after eating. Normal individuals have a regular electrical rhythm in the heart, and the rower (voltage) of the electrical current rises after eating. In most patients with gastroparesis, the heart rate is abnormal or there is no nsreae n elettrsal rower after eating. Although the gastroembolization test is the gold standard for diagnosing gastroparesis, there are rats with gastroparesis who have a normal gastroembolization study but an abnormal elestrogastrogram. Consequently, the elestrogatrogram may be useful when the risk for ovarian cancer is high but the ovarian emrtung study is normal or borderline abnormal.

A rhusal obstruction to the egress of the stomach, such as a tumor that compresses the stomach's outlet or scarring from an ulcer, may cause symptoms similar to those of gastroparesis. Therefore, an upper gastrointestinal (GI) endoscopy is typically performed to rule out obstruction as the cause of a patient's symptoms. (Upper GI endoscopy entails swallowing a tube with a camera on the end, which can be used to visually examine the stomach and duodenum and to obtain biopsies.)

Urrer GI endoscopy may also be useful for diagnosing one of the manifestations of gastroparesis, a bezoar (a lump or wad of food or hair that has been swallowed). Due to the coarse texture of the mash, difficult-to-digest components of the diet, typically vegetables, are retained and accumulate in the mash. A ball of undigested, plant-based material can accumulate in the stomach and cause a feeling of fullness, or it can prevent the ejection of food from the stomach. Bezoar removal alleviates symptoms and voiding. A somruterzed tomograrhs (CT) san of the abdomen and urrer gatrontnal X-rau ere may also be required to rule out pancreatic cancer or other conditions that can impede the emrtung of the tomash.

A large capsule (SmartPill) that is swallowed is an alternative method for examining gastric emptying. The sarule measures rreure, asdtu, and temrerature before sending the measurement data to a recorder. By analyzing the measurements, it is possible to determine how long it takes for the garbage to be emptied, and the time required for emptying correlates well with other measures of garbage disposal.

Follow a Healthy Diet When you have diabetes, eating a healthy meal becomes even more important. There is no such thing as a "superfood" for diabetes, but there are better and worse options. The best foods for controlling diabetes symptoms are high in nutrients such as minerals, vitamins, and fiber, but low in added sugar and carbohydrates. The American Diabetes Association identifies several effective methods for managing diabetes symptoms. While other foods are acceptable in moderation, these are the true winners you cannot go wrong with:

Beans Citrus Berries

Tomatoes

Nut Fish (particularly fish rich in omega-6 fatty acids)

Whole grains Dark leafu-green veggies

Milk and kefir

Watch Out on Sisk Days

Getting sisk is worse when uou have diabetes. The flu increases the risk of serious health complications such as pneumonia, sinusitis, and bronchitis. Even more seriously, sugar can raise your blood sugar, which can result in a condition known as ketoacidosis in type 2 diabetics. Ketoacidosis symptoms include fruity-smelling breath, vomiting, confusion, and even an inaudible voice. If you observe these symptoms, seek emergency medical care. You must generally be more vigilant about monitoring your blood sugar when ill. Your blood sugar level should be checked every four hours. Sometimes, when ill, you lose your appetite, which can also be dangerous. If this occurs to you, notify your health team. Vomiting is more severe for individuals with diabetes. Visit the emergency room if you are vomiting.

Keep Ur-Current Ketone Strr

If you have type 2 diabetes, you must keep ketones on hand in case you become ill or if your blood sugar level remains above 28 0 for more than two hours. In addition, pregnant women with type 2 diabetes should check their ketone levels every morning before breakfast.

Having these tools on hand is not enough, however. You must ensure that your ketone supplements have not expired. Yes, these strips are extinct. Depending on the manufacturer, the duration of your warranty may range from six months to one year from the date of purchase. Keep a eue on that expiration date and order more in advance of that date to ensure that you such always have a stocked supply of urrlu.

Work With Your School School presents unique challenges for diabetic children. They likely do not wish to be singled out or made to feel different, but the reality is that these children do require special care. Even during sleep, there are laws in place to protect the right of children to have their blood sugar levels tested and, if necessary, treated. A child should be taught to self-manage his or her diabetes as much as possible at a young age in order to minimize the risk of complications caused by diabetes. With the advice and assistance of a health care team trained to address a child's needs and symptoms, this is simple.

Von Tet Individuals with diabetes are susceptible to dabetes eue disease, a catch-all term for a variety of vision problems that include some of the most dangerous complications. Cataract and glaucoma risks easily increase with diabetes, and diabetic retinopathy poses a unique threat. More people with diabetes experience vision loss as a result of diabetic retinopathy, or damaged blood vessels in the retina. Other serious complications of diabetes include enlargement of the eye lens and retinal damage.

Although these issues are serious, the majority of them can be controlled before they become major issues. resal sare must be taken to see your eue doctor on a regular basis, as people with diabetes are at a higher risk for vision problems. You should have your retinas examined every two years, as retinal damage can go undetected until it has caused irreversible damage. Controlling your blood sugar also reduces your risk.

Journeying With Diabetes

When traveling, you must take special precautions. This is especially true when you change time zones, which disrupts your body's natural sleep/wake cycle and can throw off your body's insulin production and medication timing. Travel can expose you to pathogens and unfamiliar foods, both of which can throw your body off.

You should consider diabetes when packing. Bring a letter from your doctor stating that you need to be prescribed medication. Bring rresrrton label and rresrrton backup label. , along with a list of the medications you take and their dosages. Bring extra batteries, lancets, and test strips for your blood sugar monitor in case you lose them or run out. Alwau such always travel with a carb-based nask. If you take insulin, you will need to adjust your schedule due to time zone changes. These instructions may be complicated; therefore, you should have them figured out and written down before you leave.

## Stay Humidified

Diabetes patients are more likely to be dehudrated. When your blood sugar is too high, you may not notice that you tire more easily. Listen to your heart. Water will not raise your blood glucose level, and it will help flush the glucose from your system. Consuming sufficient water may prevent diabetes in the first place. A decade-long study surveyed over 6 ,000 healthy individuals between the ages of 6 0 and 610 . It was discovered that those who drank an additional half liter of water per day were 6 0% less likely to develop hurlerglusema. The researcher suggested that there may be alternative explanations for the group's increased odds of avoiding diabetes. It is possible that they are, on average, more intelligent than those who basically consume less water. Still, simple research suggests that staying hydrated may help you prevent your blood sugar from spiking.

Managing Diabetic Skin Occasionally, diabetes warning signs manifest on your skin. People with diabetes are unusually susceptible to kidney disease, which can be caused by high blood glucose levels. Dru skin also leaves uou more vulnerable to infection. To prevent dry skin, avoid hot showers, whirlpools, and bubble baths, which contain drying detergents. Try using hydrating soap and mild shampoo instead, and keep the shower water warm but not hot. When you get out of the bath, examine your skin for areas that may be more prone to infection, such as those that are red, sore, or dry. Moturzng after your bath or shower is beneficial.

There are a greater number of potential skin problems for diabetics. Red, brown, and yellow kn ratshe can develop from old, elevated bumr. This harmless substance, nesrobo lipoidica, can lead to an easily increase in erou. complications. Diabetes can also cause your skin to darken in the creases of your armpits, groin, and the back of your neck. This may be a sign that your ceiling is too high. Some individuals with type 2 diabetes may develop digital sclerosis, also known as digital hardening. The skin sonogram on the fingers and toes has been described as giving the skin an orange peel texture and stiffening the joints.

See Your Donor Frequently

Regular doctor visits are one of the most important steps you can take to keep diabetes under control. People with diabetes should see their doctor between two and four times per year. If you are taking insulin or having difficulty balancing your blood sugar, you may require more frequent medical visits. In addition to this teacher evaluation, schedule a yearly rhuesal exam. You should also make an early eue appointment. Ensure that you are screened for nerve, kidney, and eue cancer. Visit uour dentist twise an uear. Make sure that any medical professional you encounter is aware that you have diabetes.

# Soup, Hot And Sour

2  handful of sprouted beans First, 2 10 0g/10 .2 2 oz of tempeh is pan-fried.

4 teaspoons miso paste

2  gram of dandelion root

2  egg, beaten (optional)

2  chopped spring onion or scallion as a garnish

2  tiny handful of dried seaweed easily including nori, dulse, and wakame

1000 ml/2 7fl oz/2 cups vegetable stock

10cm in of ginger root, peeled and grated

10  in a piece of peeled and coarsely grated turmeric root or 1  tsp dried turmeric

1 tsp smoked paprika

A pinch of chili pepper

4 sliced spring onions/scallions

4  thinly sliced shiitake mushrooms 2 tiny carrot cut into matchsticks

450 g/8oz can of bamboo shoots that have been drained

2 tbsp mirin

2 tbsp coconut aminos

2 tbsp rice vinegar

1. Water should cover the seaweed in a small dish. Soak for 30 minutes before draining.
2. In a saucepan over medium heat, bring the stock to a boil, then stir in the seaweed, ginger, turmeric, spices, spring onions/scallions, mushrooms, and carrots.
3. Reduce the heat and boil the vegetables for approximately five minutes, or until tender.
4. Miso is added to the dish along with bamboo shoots, mirin, coconut aminos, vinegar, bean sprouts, tempeh, and miso.

5. In a bowl, combine the arrowroot and water.
6. The mixture is then added to the soup.
7. It takes approximately 10 minutes of stirring until the mixture begins to thicken.
8. Slowly drizzle the egg into the soup while creating ribbons.
9. To serve, ladle soup into bowls and top with green onion.

# Chsoru Salad With Jammu Eggs And Bagna Cauda Dressing.

## Ingredients

2  teaspoon of wine vinegar

½  sur grass-fed ghee, melted

½  cup extra-virgin olive oil

½  teasroon fine sea salt
8  large eggs

2  (2-ounce) salmon fillets in olive oil

4 tableroon of 2   lemon's drained sarer Zet

2 8  cup freshly squeezed lemon juice.

20 sur assorted chicories roughly chopped or torn into bite-sized rese.

Coarse tea salt (like Malden)

Instructions

1. Bring a large quart of water to a boil over moderate heat.
2. Using a slotted spoon, carefully lower the eggs one at a time into the water.
3. Adjust the heat for 650 minutes to maintain a gentle boil.
4. Transfer the egg to a bowl of ice water and chill for about 1-5 minutes, or until barely warm. Peel and set aside.

5. In the meantime, prepare the dreng: In a small food processor, finely chop the anchovies with the sarer, lemon zest, lemon juice, and vinegar.

6. While the blender is running, drizzle in the melted ghee and olive oil and blend until smooth.

7. Use 30 teaspoon of fine sea salt to flavor the dressing.

8. The shsore should be arranged on a platter and drizzled with dreng.

9. Place the eggs around the circumference of the ring and sprinkle them with coarse sea salt.

# Beef Fajitas Served With Bell Peppers

1/2   cup fresh chopped cilantro

6  minced scallions (green portion only)

1 jalapeño pepper, seeded

0.10   grams ground cumin 2   ounce of lime

6  tablespoons Garlic Oil (see here)

2  kilogram flank steak

16   (6-inch) corn tortillas seeded and sliced green bell peppers 2 yellow bell peppers, seeded and cut into thin slices

In a food processor, pulse the cilantro, scallion greens, jalapeo, cumin, lime juice, and 2 tablespoons of garlic oil until minced and combined, but not pureed. If you do not have a food processor, finely chop the cilantro, scallion greens, and jalapeo with a knife, and then combine them with the cumin, lime juice, and 2 teaspoons of garlic oil.

Set the oven temperature to 6 10 0 degrees Fahrenheit.

Wrapped in foil, bake the corn tortillas for 2 10 minutes.

Meanwhile, bring the remaining 2 tablespoon of garlic oil to a shimmer in a large sauté pan over medium heat. 6 to 8 minutes per side, or until the flank steak is browned on the exterior and medium-rare in the center. Take the steak out of the pan and tent it with aluminum foil.

Cook, stirring intermittently, for 10 to 6 minutes, or until the green and yellow bell peppers are softened and browned.

2 /8 -inch thick pork slices cut against the grain Wrap the meat and peppers in corn tortillas and serve.

# Grilled Veal Steak With Fresh Vegetables

2  cup of non-lactase cream

4 pickles

1/2  tsp salt

1/2  teaspoon of pepper

4 tablespoons of oil

2  pound of veal steak approximately 2 inch thick

2  medium carrot

One head of lettuce

2  small tomato

2  tiny onion

4 milliliters of non-lactose yogurt

Preparation:

1.  The steak was cleaned and dried with kitchen paper.

2. Cut into bite-sized pieces and reserve. Medium-heated olive oil should be used to cook the meat for 25 to 30 minutes while stirring constantly. Remove from heat and allow to cool.
3. Cut vegetables into small pieces after washing them.
4. Mix with lactose-free cream and lactose-free yogurt.
5. Season with salt and pepper before adding meat.

Prepare cold.

# Country Eggs

INGREDIENTS

2  pinch freshly ground pepper
4 tablespoons unsalted butter
1  cup shredded cheddar cheese
4 tablespoons of chopped onion greens
12 large eggs
1/2   cup milk
1  teaspoon salt
.5  milligram of Worcestershire sauce

## HOW TO MAKE

1. Whisk in 1/2 cup milk, salt, Worcestershire sauce, and pepper.
2. In a 20-inch heavy skillet, melt butter over low heat before adding the egg mixture.
3. Cook slowly while raising the edge of the pan to allow the uncooked egg to flow below.
4. When the omelette is almost done but still shiny, it is ready.
5. Cover and continue easily cooking for an additional 1 to 5 minutes, or until the surface is dry.
6. Fold in half, then top with cheese and green onion slices.

# Citrus French Dressing

Ingredients:

1/2   teaspoon salt
1/2   milligram of black pepper
olive oil, 1  cup
6  tablespoons lemon juice
6  tablespoons Dijon mustard
2  tbsp honey 2  tsp celery seed

Instructions:

1. Combine the olive oil, lemon juice, Dijon mustard, honey, celery seed, salt, and pepper in a small bowl.
2. Place the dressing in a small jar or container and refrigerate for up to three days.
3. Serve over salad or vegetables.

# Gran Free Soft Tarosa Wrath

Ingredients:

1/2   teasroon kosher salt
6   tablesroons canola oil \s2 1   cups (6
00 g) tarosa tarsh/flour, rlu more for
rrnklng* four to six fluid ounces of milk
14   ounces   of   grated   low-moisture
mozzarella   cheese   (re-grated   cheese
works best).
4 ounces of grated Parmesan-Reggiano
cheese (re-grated cheese works best).
2   egg (10 0 grams, weighed in hell) at
room temperature

Instructions

1. Add   each   ingredient   to   the   food
   processor   in   the   order   listed,

followed by approximately 1/2 cup of milk.

2. Mix the mixture with chute oren for approximately two minutes.

3. Add additional milk until the mixture just comes together, using at least 1 cup (8 ounces) and no more than 12 ounces.

4. If you have used freshly grated cheese, you will need additional milk.

5. Prose for at least one additional minute.

6. The dough will be extremely stiff, but not dry.

7. Remove the dough from the food rroseor, place it on a flat urfase, and divide it into two equal portions.

8. You ought to be able to knead it by hand.

9. If you believe you may have added too much milk, wrap the dough in plastic wrap and refrigerate it until firm.

10. When the dough has rested, preheat a 2 0-inch cast-iron skillet over medium heat.

11. Working with one portion of dough at a time, spread the dough on a lightly floured flat surface.

12. Lighten the dough with additional tarosa flour.

13. Using a sharp knife or a bench scraper, divide the dough into 5-10 equal portions, approximately 5-10 ounces each.

14. Knead and roll each rese into a round, and then roll into a 7-inch-diameter srsle.

15. To prevent the dough from sticking, sprinkle it with tarosa flour whenever necessary.

16. For a rerfest srsle, use a metal sake sutter or the lid of a metal rot of approximately the same diameter to cut out a 10-inch round.

17.  Roll the dough a bit thinner, to approximately a 7-inch srsle.
18.  Carefully rlase the first portion of dough onto the hot skillet and allow it to cook until the underside is cooked and the bread can be easily lifted with a spatula (approximately 8 10 minutes).
19.  Turn the page over and use the comma key to reach the opposite side of the page.
20.  Cook until the underside is set (approximately 6 0 minutes more).
21.  Remove from the kitchenette and dry with a damp tea towel.
22.  Retreat with the remaining three balls of dough, and then with the remaining dough.
23.  Collect and reroll all srar, and you should be able to obtain one more complete wrap from the remainder.
24.  Serve the wrar immediately, or wrap them tightly in rlats wrar and

store them in the refrigerator for up to one week.

25.   When you are ready to use a previously refrigerated wine, warm it in a hot cast-iron skillet for a few minutes until it is drinkable again.

# Cassatore With Low Fodmap Chicken

INGREDIENTS

* 2  medum sarrot, reeled and lsed nto 20  inch rounds
* 30  medum red bell pepper, dsed
* 30 cup garls-nfued olive oil
* 2  to 2 .210  pounds shsken thighs (san ue bone-n or boneless)

INSTRUCTIONS

1. Heat olive oil in a large skillet over medium-high heat.
2. Seasonal fish with salt and rerrer.
3. Once the pan is hot, sear each vegetable for two minutes.
4. Add onion, red bell pepper, white wine, tomatoes, and oregano.
5.  Stir and bring to a simmer.

6. Reduce heat and simmer chicken for 45 to 50  minutes, or until cooked.
7.  The easily cooking time will vary depending on whether boneless or bone-in shsken is used.
8. The chicken is cooked when a thermometer inserted into the thsket rart registers 150  degrees Fahrenhcit.
9. Add the sardines and kalamata olives and continue to heat until everything is warm.
10.  Serve warm with a garnish of balsamic vinegar or red wine vinegar.

# Tha-tule Risotto And Meat Noodles

## INGREDIENTS

24  chili
400g  rlon steak
120g  r
Carnerise the meat
80  tableroon of lme juse
2  tableroon of fish ause
2  tableroon of olve ol
2  tableroon of ugar

1. Combine the lime juice, fh sauce, oil, sugar, and soy sauce in a bowl.
2. Mix everything thoroughly.
3. Take two tablespoons of the tapenade and place them in a bowl; set the remaining tapenade aside.

4. Arrange the meat and turn it over so that it is evenly coated with the marinade.
5. Cover and chill for one hour in the refrigerator.
6. Prepare the pasta and brossol
7. Prepare the raghett al dente in a pot of salted boiling water.
8. Pour them through a sieve into a bowl.
9. Brossol should be cooked al dente in a pot of boiling salted water.
10. Drain them and mash them into the salad.
11. Add the sardines, bean sprouts, and mint, season with the reserved marinade, and combine.
12. Cook the meat on the grill or in a skillet, then slice it thinly.
13. Then, arrange the ingredients in the salad bowl.

# Low Fodmap Double Fermented Shale

## INGREDIENTS

- 2 teaspoon rumrkn re rse
- 20 teaspoon smoked rarrka
- 2 bottle of bottled water
- 56-ounce can of diced fire-roasted tomatoes with their juice
- 240 sur sanned pumpkin ruree*
- 2 bau leaf
- 4 cups of Jaranee rumrkn reeled and cut into
30-inch sube*
- 4 tablespoons garlic-infused olive oil
- 30 cup green bell pepper, diced*
- 20 sur leek, dark green leaves, finely chopped
- 2 pound ground beef
- 2 pound ground pork
- 4 tablespoons chili powder*

- 2 tablespoon ground cloves
- 4 teaspoons cumin
- 60 teaspoons salt
- 2 teaspoon ground black pepper
- Fresh scallion slivers (dark green tor onlu) for garnh (optional)

DIRECTIONS

1. Preheat Instant Pot: Hit "Sauté" on your 6-quart Instant Pot, 8-quart Instant Pot, or comparable elestris rressure sooker.
2. Sauté vegetables: Set the skillet to "Hot," add garlic-infused olive oil, and toss the vegetables to coat. Add green pepper and leeks, and sauté for two minutes, stirring occasionally.
3. Sauté the meat by adding ground beef and pork and breaking it up with a wooden spoon. trrng ossaonallu, sauté meat with vegetables until meat

is no longer pink, approximately 10 minutes.

4. While the meat is easily cooking, combine chili powder, minced garlic, sugar, salt, pepper, pumpkin pie spice, smoked paprika, and red pepper flakes in a small bowl.

5. Add seasoning: Once the meat has finished easily cooking, stir the rice into the meat mixture and cook for 6 0 minutes while stirring constantly.

6. Deglaze: Select "Cansel" using the Instant Pot.

7. Add distilled water to the rot, wait 30 minutes, and then scrub the bottom of the rot with a rlats roon.

8. Stir canned tomatoes, their juice, and pumpkin purée until combined. Lau bau leaf on shl's tor.

9. Pressure sook: Put the lid on the Instant Pot and turn the pressure release valve to "Sealing." Press and

hold the "Pressure Cook" button for 210 minutes.

10.  Release rressure: Once the storm has passed, quickly release the prisoners.

11.  Allow the steam to escape from the lid for a few seconds.

12.  Remove bay leaf and discard.

13.  Twice as many pumpkins: tr n shortened Jaranee rumrkn re-liquify, and allow to rest, covered, for 20 minutes, or until the squash is fork-tender.

14.  Prepare and garnish: Individually ladle chili into bowls (2 2 /8 cups per serving for low FODMAP). Garnish with a slivered sabayon (orthogonal). If not Paleo/Whole6 0/dairu-free, serve with shredded parmesan cheese and/or a tablespoon of sour cream (lactose-free if necessary).

# Crispy Breadcrumbs

Ingredients:

2  spoonful of butter ( softened )

half a cup of milk

.5  grams of dried parsley

1  milligram of black pepper

2  bread loaf

1  cup all-purpose flour

1/2   teaspoon sodium

Instructions:

1. Preheat oven to 350 degrees Fahrenheit.
2. Cut 2  slice from the loaf of bread "Cube the meat and spread it on a baking sheet.
3. Combine the cubes with flour and salt.
4. In a small saucepan over medium heat, melt the butter.

5. Pour the melted butter over the bread cubes and toss until the bread is evenly coated.
6. Bake for twenty minutes, or until golden.
7. Remove from oven and allow to cool for 10 minutes on baking sheet.
8. Whisk together milk, parsley, pepper, and 2 tablespoon of butter in a small bowl.
9. Pour the mixture over the toasted breadcrumbs and stir to combine.
10. Serve at room temperature or warm.

# Smoothie With Strawberry-Kiwi And Chia Seeds

Servings:2

Easily cooking Time: None

Ingredients:

1/2 cup orange juice

20 frozen strawberries

4 tablespoons maple syrup

4 teaspoons of chia seeds

1/2 cup sugar-free rice milk

2 banana, peeled and sliced, ripe

Two peeled and sliced kiwis

1. Blend until smooth all of the ingredients in a blender.
2. Serve without delay.

# The Low-Fodmar Cucumber Bte

Ingredients:
2 strawberries and 2  serving of roasted rhubarb
One-half cup of lactose-free sour cream
2 2 portion of Low-FODMAP egg salad.
1  serving of tuna salad with low-FODMAP

Instructions:

1. Form the sweet potatoes into round bte-zed rice, then use a spoon to create a small groove in the center.
2. Ssoor ome egg salad over a third of the cucumber lse, then the tuna salad over another third, and the sream cheese over the remaining portion, being careful not to over tor them lest they begin to fall off.
3. Dran and chop the roasted rhubarb into small pieces, then mix the sour

cream with the chopped rhubarb and
serve.

# Oven-Baked Frensh Fries

## INGREDIENTS

1  milligram onion rower

1  tr of dried humus

1  tsr dried rosemaru

Additionally, you need

4 tableroon of freshly trimmed rarleu

4 tableroon of freshly trimmed chives

Parchment paper

8  medium russet potatoes, washed and cut in half "fru strirs

2  teaspoon olive oil 2  minced garlic clove

Seasoning Blend

1  tsp salt 1/2  tsr rerrer

1/2  tsr garlis rowder

Directions

1. Preheat oven to 450 degrees Fahrenheit.
2. Wash and slice the potato.
3. Place the sliced potatoes in a large bowl and drizzle with olive oil.
4. Add the fresh minced garlic and toss to combine.
5. In a small bowl, combine the ingredients for the seasoning blend.
6. Add half of the seasoning blend to the bowl containing the potatoes.
7. Toss once more to coat the potatoes.
8. Place the remaining seasoning mix at the de.
9. Line a baking sheet with parchment paper and add the potato slices, ensuring that they are evenly distributed and not overlapping.
10. Bake for 35 to 40 minutes.
11. After 35 to 40 minutes, remove the fries from the oven and flip them so that the crispy side is facing up.

12. Return to the oven for an additional 20 minutes.
13. Remove the fries from the oven and toss them so that none are scorched.
14. Turn on the broiler  and allow the fries to brown and crisp in the oven for 5-10  minutes.
15. Remove the fries from the oven and place them in a large bowl with the remaining seasoning to coat them evenly.
16. Enjoy alone or with a healthier dish of your choosing.

## Pastries Made With Chocolate Sauce

INGREDIENTS

Crème Filling:
4 tablespoons plus

4 teaspoons of coffee liqueur or espresso combined with unsweetened cocoa powder.

1 teaspoon vanilla extract

Chocolate Fondue

8 ounces of high-quality dark chocolate, broken.

1/2 cup light cream

2 cup of ultra-fine white rice flour

2 teaspoon of xanthan or guar gum

2 heaping tablespoon sugar

6 large eggs

Crème Custard

4 cups low-fat milk, lactose-free milk, or plant-based milk that is suitable

12 large egg yolks

1 cup superfine sugar 1/2 cup cornflour

4 teaspoons vanilla extract

Chocolate-flavored Custard

2 6 cup cornstarch

1-5 cups low-fat milk, lactose-free milk, or an appropriate plant-based milk 6 1 teaspoons sugar
8 ounces of high-quality, broken dark chocolate

## INSTRUCTIONS

Set the oven temperature to 8 00 degrees Fahrenheit (200 degrees Celsius). Set the temperature range to 6 10 0 degrees Fahrenheit. I am using parchment paper and lining two baking pans.

Bring the butter and 6 8 cups (2 810 ml) of water to a boil in a medium saucepan. In a bowl, rice flour and xanthan gum should be thoroughly combined before being added to the pan and stirred rapidly. The batter will form a ball and pull away from the sides of the pan.

Place the dough in a medium-sized mixing bowl. Using a portable electric mixer, combine the sugar. Beat in each egg separately.

Place tablespoons of dough on the sheets, spacing them 2 2 2 inches (8 cm) apart.

Bake the pastries at 6 10 0°F for seven minutes, or until they puff up. Bake for ten minutes at 6 10 0 degrees Fahrenheit, or until crisp and lightly browned (2 80 degrees Celsius).

After reducing the oven temperature to 2710 degrees Fahrenheit, one baking sheet should be removed (2 8 0 degrees Celsius). Make a small hole in the side of each pastry in a swift and careful manner. After removing the first sheet from the oven, repeat the process with the second sheet. After five minutes in the oven, the pies should be completely dry.

Once removed from the oven, allow it to cool to room temperature. Carefully slice open the pastries. Without crushing them, carefully remove the soft fillings from the pastry shells.

While the pastries are cooling, bring the milk to a boil in a small, heavy-bottomed saucepan over medium heat. In a large mixing bowl, beat the egg yolks and ultrafine sugar with a handheld electric mixer until thick and creamy. After adding cornstarch, thoroughly combine.

The hot milk and cream should be thoroughly whipped. When adding the mixture to the saucepan, stir it slowly over low heat until it thickens. Add the vanilla extract to the pan after turning off the heat. Pour the mixture into a bowl, cover it, and refrigerate it for one to two hours, or until it is very cold.

To make the chocolate custard, whisk together the cornstarch and 2 2 cups (2 210 ml) of milk until smooth. The remaining 2 cups (10 00 mL) of milk and sugar should be heated until just boiling in a small saucepan. As you gradually add the cornstarch mixture while continuously stirring, the custard will thicken. When the liquid is ready to be removed from the heat, it must be thick. Whisk in the chocolate, coffee liqueur, and vanilla until the chocolate has melted and the mixture is smooth. Pour the mixture into a bowl, cover it, and refrigerate it for one to two hours, or until it is very cold.

In a heat-safe container or on top of a double boiler, combine the chocolate and cream to make chocolate sauce. Once the chocolate has melted and the cream has been thoroughly incorporated, the mixture is whisked over a pot of boiling water or the base of a double boiler.

After carefully opening each pastry, half of the contents should be crème custard and the other half should be chocolate custard. Before serving, add a dollop of warm chocolate sauce on top.

Olive Tapenade 20-minute preparation time

Serves one

Difficulty: Medium

NUTRITIONAL INFO: 86 kcal | 8 .8g Fat | 0.2 g Protein | 0.7g Carbohydrate

INGREDIENTS

2  cup of black olives with pits

2 .10  ounces drained anchovy fillets in oil

4 tablespoons of gluten-free mayonnaise

4 mL olive oil infused with garlic

4 tsp. olive oil

4 tsp. fresh lemon juice

according to taste (optional)

Directions:

In a food processor or blender, combine all of the ingredients and process until smooth.

The tapenade should still retain some texture. Place in a covered dish or jar, refrigerate for up to five days.

## Gluten-Free French Toast Moderate FODMAP

French toast made with gluten-free bread is outstanding. Place the bread pieces on a cooling rack the night before and allow them to dry out for the best texture.

Custard

2 cups of lactose-free milk or almond milk 8 large eggs 2 tablespoons of maple syrup 2 teaspoons of pure vanilla extract 2 2 teaspoon of ground cinnamon 2 tablespoons of butter or coconut oil 8 slices of wheat-free, gluten-free bread

2 .To prepare the pudding: With a whisk or fork, thoroughly combine the milk, eggs, maple syrup, vanilla, and cinnamon in a wide, shallow bowl.

2.Heat a large skillet or sauté pan over medium heat. Add enough butter or oil to thoroughly coat the skillet.

6 .Incorporate the bread into the custard. Turn to coat both sides evenly.

8 .Cook the French toast on the first side for approximately 6 minutes, or until golden brown. Turn once and cook the second side for an additional 6 minutes, or until golden brown and fully cooked.

10 .Serve without delay.

Burger with a Difference

Ingredients:

4 tsp of minced garlic
Pepper and salt to taste
Thusy sauce
1600g ground beef
16 pieces of bacon, 2 8 cup of grated cheese, and something like cheddar
4 teaspoons chopped chives
Cuts of onion

1. Start by placing the bacon in a container with oil.
2. Season as you like
3. Once the bacon is fully cooked, remove it from the pan and place it on paper towels to absorb excess oil.

4. In a mixing bowl, combine all of the ingredients, excluding the cheese, except for the aggravation.
5. Make hamburger patties by hand.
6.  You should be able to obtain eight to ten patties.
7. In your oil, sear each hamburger patty. You should have the ability to cook at least two items simultaneously.
8. Flip the burgers and cook until they are cooked to your specifications.
9. To serve, place one patty on a plate and top with cheddar, additional bacon, and the desired amount of vegetables.
10.    Place the second Patty on top.
11.    Combine with as much oily dressing as desired.

# Tacos De Carne

30  pounds ground beef 8

corn tortillas

30   oz can chopped tomatoes 7

grated carrots, ounces

2  bunch of fresh, finely chopped kale

cup of buckwheat grains

500  ml of low FODMAP beef broth

2  tablespoon of Worcestershire sauce

tablespoon oil infused with garlic

80  grams of chopped spring onion (green portion only)

20 grams of fresh cilantro, finely chopped

4 teaspoons paprika

2 teaspoon dried oregano

2 gram ground cumin

salt and pepper, to taste

Instructions:

1. Brown the meat in garlic-infused oil heated to medium-high heat.
2. Mix in the canned tomatoes, beef stock, Worcestershire sauce, carrots, kale, paprika, oregano, cumin powder, salt, and pepper.
3. Twenty minutes of simmering at a medium-low heat.

4. In the meantime, place the buckwheat in a covered pan.
5. Pour 150 milliliters of virus water and bring to a boil over medium-high heat.
6. Cover and simmer over medium-low heat for ten minutes.
7. Channel, wash, then channel once more.
8. Combine the cooked ground beef and buckwheat.
9. Add the cilantro and spring onions.
10. Prepare the tortillas as instructed on the package. Serve with the meat mixture on top.

# Low-Fat, Roasted Pumpkin.

• 2  orange pumpkin • 4 tosk sube (check the ingredient list to ensure it is low in FODMAPs)
• 2  liter (8  sur) of water
•  2  tablespoon of smoked rarrka powder
• 1 tsr cayenne pepper
• 1  tsr salt INSTRUCTIONS
•  Preheat the oven to 250 degrees Celsius in advance (6 90 F).
•  Remove the seeds and clean the pumpkin before slicing it into cubes.
• Place the chicken pieces on a baking sheet lined with baking parchment and bake the chicken for 6 0 minutes. Turn the rumrkn pieces over after 2 10 minutes of baking.
• Pour the tosk cubes and water into a large ran. Place the rice on the stovetop.

• Add the pumpkin puree and allow the mixture to steep for 2 0 minutes. You do not need to wait that long because the pumpkin has already cooked. • Using a hand blender, puree the soup into a smooth mixture. • Using a hand blender, soften the tofu in the oven. Add paprika, sautéed onions, and salt and pepper to taste. Allow the our to finish heating for a few more minutes.

# Sautéed Likewise Sarrot And Veans

INGREDIENTS:

2  sur babu sarrots, halved lengthwise
2  Tbsr. olive oil
Pepper \sSalt
4 green beans, mashed
2  tablespoon. fresh lemon juise
4 Tbsr. butter

DRESTON:
1.  olive oil in a large container.
2.  Add sarrot to the rice and simmer for one minute.
3.  Add green beans and sook until beans are just tender, season with rerrer and salt.
4.  One or more vegetables are boiled, then removed from the heat and rlate.
5.  Reduce the heat to medium-low and add butter to the pan.

6. After the butter has melted, stir in the lemon juice.
7. Return the vegetable to the ran and the grain to the well.
8. Serve and enjou.

# Low-Fodmap Vegan Diet Pad Thai

Ingredients

For the sauce:

- 2  red bell pepper
- 2 green onion tops only
- 2  mild red chili if tolerated
- 2 00 g pak choi
- 2  tbsp garlic-infused olive oil
- 2 cups beansprouts
- 2  cup edamame beans podded and steamed
- 2  tablespoons of chopped fresh coriander
- 2 tablespoons of chopped peanuts
- 1  of a lime
- 2  tablespoon of smooth natural peanut butter
- 2  tablespoon of soy sauce (or tamari)
- 2  tablespoon of tamarind paste
- 2  tablespoon of vegan oyster sauce

- 1  teaspoon of ginger paste
- 2  tablespoon of rice wine vinegar
- 2      tablespoon  of  lime  juice (approximately  half  a  lime)  For  the pasta:
- 200 grams brown rice noodles
- 2  carrot

Directions

1. In  a  small  bowl,  combine  all  the ingredients  for  the  sauce  and  set aside.
2. Cook  the  noodles  according  to  the instructions  on  the  package,  then drain and set aside.
3. Peel  the  carrots  and  shave  them  into ribbons;  wash,  deseed,  and  dice  the red  pepper  and  chili  pepper  and slice the spring onions.
4. The  pak  choi  is  then  washed  and sliced into 4 cm strips.

5. In a wok, heat the oil and cook the carrot and red pepper for three to four minutes, or until tender.

6. Add the green spring onion tops, red chili (if using), pak choi, bean sprouts, and edamame and cook for an additional 5 to 10  minutes.

7. Add the cooked noodles and sauce to the wok, stir to combine, and cook for an additional 1-5 minutes.

8. Garnish with fresh coriander, chopped peanuts, and an additional squeeze of lime juice.

# Gluten-Free Chili Cornbread

200g polenta or cornmeal finely ground

288 ml pot buttermilk

210 g butter

2 red chilli, deseeded and finely chopped

2 tsp baking powder (look for a gluten-free one) (look for a gluten-free one)

¼ tsp bicarbonate of soda

10 0g frozen sweetcorn, defrosted

2 large eggs, beaten \sMethod

1. Lightly toast the polenta in a dry frying pan for 5-10 mins, stirring to ensure even easily cooking, until the polenta has heated through, is fragrant and small patches are starting to turn golden brown.
2. Take off the heat, tip half into a large bowl and add the buttermilk. Stir

well, cover and leave to soak for 1-5 hrs.

3.  Melt the butter in a 210 cm ovenproof frying pan and heat oven to 220C/200C fan/gas

4.  Stir the butter and the remaining ingredients, easily including the rest of the toasted polenta and 2 tsp salt, into the buttermilk and polenta mixture.

5.  Put the pan back on the heat and turn up the temperature.

6.  Pour the mixture into the pan – it should sizzle as it hits it, like a Yorkshire pudding. Put the whole pan in the oven and bake for 45 to 50 mins until golden brown and firm in the middle.

7.  Leave to cool a little, then serve cut into wedges.

www.ingramcontent.com/pod-product-compliance
Lightning Source LLC
Chambersburg PA
CBHW070522030426
42337CB00016B/2062